YOUR KNOWLEDGE HAS VALUE

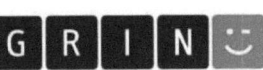

Integrative Literature Review on the Importance of Cultural Competence in Nursing

Gabby Ian

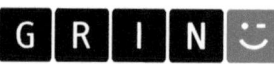

Bibliographic information published by the German National Library:

The German National Library lists this publication in the National Bibliography; detailed bibliographic data are available on the Internet at http://dnb.dnb.de.

ISBN: 9783346503800
This book is also available as an ebook.

© GRIN Publishing GmbH
Nymphenburger Straße 86
80636 München

Print and binding: Books on Demand GmbH, Norderstedt, Germany
Printed on acid-free paper from responsible sources.

The present work has been carefully prepared. Nevertheless, authors and publishers do not incur liability for the correctness of information, notes, links and advice as well as any printing errors.

GRIN web shop: https://www.grin.com/document/1044995

Importance of Cultural Competence in Nursing

Integrative Literature Review on the Importance of Cultural Competence in Nursing

Abstract

The Nursing profession has been established as one of the dynamic and evolving fields that involve interactions with healthcare professionals and patients from diverse backgrounds. The rising multicultural society and diversities call for nursing practitioners to prepare and get ready to deliver quality care and patient outcomes to every patient irrespective of their socio-economic status, color, ethnicity, or race differentiations (Kaihlanen, Hietapakka & Heponiemi, 2019). This target can only be achieved when nurses are trained on attending to all patients equally without prejudice and working in a multicultural society without any discrimination. This should begin from the core units where nurses are getting trained, especially in medical schools early enough so that when they finally get to work, they have the capacity to handle and work across different cultures and diverse backgrounds while maintaining respect for everyone regardless of the existing differences between them (Douglas et al., 2014). In this regard, this paper seeks to conduct a critical literature review on the importance of cultural competence in the nursing profession.

Integrative Literature Review on the Importance of Cultural Competence in Nursing

Introduction

According to Sharifi, Adib-Hajbaghery, and Najafi (2019), nurses have been on the front line for a long time to deliver care to a variety of patients drawn from diverse backgrounds. Most nurses have realized that providing care in the nursing profession, especially in a culturally competent manner, is essential. This is considering that it ensures that every patient receives the right treatment, equal, and quality healthcare without being discriminated against based on their socio-economic differences, ethnicity, race, or color (Loftin et al., 2013). This characteristic is critical for nurses because it enables them to assess, diagnose, and to treat patients with the best interventions for quality health outcomes and quality care. In the absence of cultural competence in the nursing profession, some nurses may find themselves favoring some patients over others by giving them special attention compared to others. This might result when some clients are perceived to be economically stable compared to others or because they might be coming from the same ethnic background (Reyes, Hadley & Davenport, 2013).

Discrimination in the field of nursing can only result in increased mortality rates and more morbidities, especially in cases when nurses fail to give equal attention to all patients. In the contemporary world and current society, the most nurse has been working in different backgrounds and settings from where they grew and were brought up, and this explains the significance of training nurses to have a good understanding of the importance of diverse backgrounds, respect for culture, and diversity (Cai, 2016). Therefore creating the attitude of cultural awareness in the nursing field can be the best approach and strategy towards reducing the impacts and consequences of having a nurse who is not culturally competent. In this regard, this paper seeks to provide an integrative literature review on the importance ensuring cultural competence in nursing profession.

4

Background of the Study

According to Almutairi, McCarthy, and Gardner (2015), nurses who lack cultural awareness cannot be culturally competent to care for a wide range of patients. They might leave them unattended as they concentrate on those with whom they share the same skin color, language, race, or ethnic background. This is potentially dangerous because the lives of the other discriminated patients are left at stake, and anything can happen to them. Douglas et al. (2014) pinpoint that critically ill patients can experience increased stress, which can only deteriorate their health further. The nurse's role to care by washing, grooming, feeding, and giving medications to patients might also not be accomplished in good time, and this also affects the healing process, and it takes longer than expected. It is also important to note that a prolonged healing process increases the length of stay in the hospital, and this increases the cost of health care (Loftin et al., 2013).

Some of the patients might not be able to pay for the bills because they are not economically stable. This shows that being culturally competent for nurses is the basis of providing quality care for all, which will fasten the healing process, and this will reduce the length of stay, and less money will be paid to the hospital (Sharifi, Adib-Hajbaghery & Najafi, 2019). However, not all nurses are culturally competent, and this requires urgent intervention. Lack of awareness, especially in intensive care units, can contribute to high mortality rates since most of the patients require urgent care.

Problem Statement

According to Jeffreys (2016), cultural competence enables nurses to work effectively in the context of difference. They become conversant with how to relate with patients from different cultures, respect them, manage diversity, and be sensitive when delivering care. However, this has not been the case, and some nurses are never sensitive about diversity and culture. This can even get worse in case a nurse has negative attitudes toward a certain race, ethnic group, or people of

5

certain skin color (Cai, 2016). This can lower patient safety and lead to high mortalities. Developing a curriculum that trains nursing students on how to handle patients from different backgrounds can reduce the negative outcome related to this problem (Almutairi, McCarthy & Gardner, 2015).

Purpose of the Study

This study aims to give insight and understanding of the importance of developing and fostering cultural competence in the nursing profession through a critical literature review of different available resource materials. At the same time, it will highlight the impacts and importance of creating a nursing curriculum that demonstrates respect for culture by equipping the nursing learners with the right attitudes, behaviors, and skills that can assist them in working with different clients from diverse backgrounds (Douglas et al., 2014). It thus seeks to analyses the concept of cultural competence through the lens of its importance in the nursing profession towards ensuring that different patients are treated and handled equally at all times without discrimination based on different factors. In this regard, the study will be guided by the following research objectives:

- Demonstrate the importance of fostering the culture of cultural competence among nursing professionals.
- Examine whether cultural competence and its components are effectively incorporated in the current and existing nursing curriculum.
- Analyze some of the possible outcomes following the nursing training to work on patients' needs from diverse backgrounds.
- Establish and demonstrate the significance of cultural competence, respect, and tolerance in the nursing profession towards ensuring quality care and improved patient outcomes.

Literature Review

In nursing, cultural competence means having the ability to care for patients who are from different backgrounds socially, economically, and culturally. Sharifi, Adib-Hajbaghery & Najafi (2019) define culture as a people's way of living. Different cultures have different ways of living, including their way of dressing, cooking, and interacting with other people. There is a variation between cultures, and the nurses need to understand these variations and care for patients while respecting all aspects of their patients' cultures. Douglas et al. (2014) define cultural diversity as the differences between the norms and values of a culture. On the other hand, cultural competence is a set of attitudes, behaviors, and policies that are expected to be part of the healthcare system, usually among the nursing profession. They enable nurses to work across a wide range of cultures effectively. Cultural competence is a component that improves the health outcomes of the patients, nurses, and health care systems (Gallagher & Polanin, 2015).

Sharifi, Adib-Hajbaghery & Najafi (2019) further contend that nursing's cultural issues are also interrelated with the socio-economic issues and the political issues in nursing. Cultural competence helps in striking a balance between culture, socio-economic issues, and political issues of nursing. The socio-economic issues in nursing include, for example, the ability of a patient from a different social-economic background to pay for their hospital bill. It is common that some of the minority and marginalized groups cannot pay for the hospital bills because they earn little or no income at all (Loftin et al., 2013). The relationship between cultural competence and the socio-economic issues is that nurses might refuse to treat patients if they cannot pay for the services. However, culturally competent nurses should be ready to treat the patients even with no money and make payment plans later after they are healed (Reyes, Hadley & Davenport, 2013). This shows respect for human life because they save the patient's life, which is their main role.

7

Reyes, Hadley & Davenport (2013) contemplates that some of the political issues of nursing that are related to cultural competence include the formulation of nursing policies, nursing staffing, and nursing salaries and remunerations. Although not directly related to the provision of care to patients, they, in one way or another, affect the execution of roles by nurses. For example, in case the nurse leaders involved in setting the amount of salaries for nurses favor one race over the others, the discriminated group can suspend or down their tools, which affects the health of the patients (Kaihlanen, Hietapakka & Heponiemi, 2019). In the medical schools, the development of cultural competence training curriculum will be a good direction in establishing a positive nursing profession about working in a cross-cultural setting while having respect for all people involved regardless of the differences. This will promote cultural safety because it ensures that there is greater equity in all the nursing activities (Garneau & Pepin, 2015).

The focus on the root cause of the problem will benefit the health care systems since there will be integration between all the cultures involved. Jeffreys (2016) explains that the federal, state, and local governments can work closely with the nursing schools to plan and implement a curriculum that will understand the nurses. The curriculum can focus on cultural awareness, cultural equity, respect for diversity, human rights, and care delivery across a multifaceted cultural landscape (Gallagher & Polanin, 2015). The curriculum should focus on the core building blocks of cultural competence such as cultural desire, encounter, skills, knowledge, and awareness. The learners need to be evaluated vigorously on different examples and case studies involving cultural competence in nursing (Jeffreys, 2016). Some good cases examples include applauding strengths and individuality and valuing individuals, empathizing with patients at all times, not judging or disregarding patient's religious backgrounds and beliefs, and speaking in terms that patients can comprehend.

According to the study conducted by Loftin et al., (2013), cultural competence is essential for the growth and development of nurses besides helping incorporate relevant societal values. This is significant considering that nursing is a versatile profession that entails taking care for the elderly, providing treatment plans, and caring for the sick from different backgrounds. The best nurses are therefore those who are technically sounds and at the same time recognized as experts in cultural competence (Loftin et al., 2013). According to their study, cultural competence is the ability of healthcare workers and nurses in general to offer their best primary care to different clients while demonstrating cultural awareness for their values, race, and beliefs. This implies that the nurses understand the patient's cultural diversity while offering care (Cai, 2016). In this connection, cultural competence is significant in nursing because it prepares nurses to attend more profoundly to their patients, relate more to patient and empathize with their patients. Patients often develop a positive feeling and positive response to treatment when they have someone who understands their unique background or speaks their language on their care team. This makes them relax and respond positively to treatment thereby leading to greater therapy and overall care. The same research contends that cultural competence is essential because it helps nurses interact, communicate, and understand different people effectively (Kratzke & Bertolo, 2013). Cultural competence more specifically centers around ensuring positive attitude, developing communication skills, acquiring knowledge of different cultural practices, and understanding the connection between patients and nurses.

Cultural competence in nursing comprises of the knowledge and skills that all nurses must possess for them to provide effective care for patients from different cultural backgrounds. The usability and application of these attitudes, knowledge, and skills are significant among nurses operating in multi cultured and cross culture societies (Cai, 2016). Besides, cultural competence is important in nursing profession considering that nursing practitioners deals with and handle patients from different cultures and backgrounds. It is therefore paramount for nurses to embrace transcultural practices and skills. This will entail understanding cultural beliefs, age, religion, sexual orientation, ethnicity, and race among other personal traits of different clients they are responsible for their primary care (Kratzke & Bertolo, 2013). According to research, cultural competence encompasses three major components including cultural awareness, cultural sensitivity, and cultural knowledge. The combination of these basic components in conjunction with practical skills and expertise, nurses can effectively offer specialized and improved primary care to diverse clients (Garneau & Pepin, 2015).

Methods with Discussion and Analysis

Methodology

The study will be based primarily on a critical literature review of different resource materials on cultural competence in the nursing profession and its importance in the field. Both quantitative and qualitative data will be utilized in this study to give a clear picture and overview of the importance of cultural competence in the nursing profession. The secondary data will be collected from peer-reviewed articles, journal publications, and other reputable websites on the importance of cultural competence in nursing. The collected data and resource materials will comprise of both qualitative and quantitative research. However, since quantifying cultural competence might be difficult because it comprises behaviors and values, the study will heavily borrow and rely on qualitative resource materials. The inclusion criteria that will be used when searching for this resource materials is that they must be based on cultural competence in nursing profession and must not be more than eight years old.

Results and Findings

Cultural competence can be defined as the ability of healthcare providers to provide services that respect and recognize their patients' social beliefs and cultural practices. Cultural competency is essential in healthcare settings since it helps in improving the quality of care and also improving the outcomes (Reyes, Hadley & Davenport, 2013). It is also vital in eliminating racial and ethnic preferences. Culture is compassionate since it influences how nurses and patients think about illness. Many opportunities and challenges in creating and delivering culturally competent services are emerging in healthcare settings due to the nation's increasing diversity (Douglas et al., 2014). Nurses' role in the healthcare system is significant since they are the first and the last point of contact with the patients.

From the numerous resource materials, it is apparent that cultural competence "guides the nurse in understanding behaviors and planning appropriate approaches to patient needs (Montenery, et al., 2013". Therefore, cultural competence is extremely important in healthcare. By understanding a patient's cultural background, an effective nurse-patient relationship can be established through the patient's right care and understanding. Furthermore, each culture has a different nursing need (Gallagher & Polanin, 2015). Similarly, the research indicated that strong leadership is essential when it comes to nursing. This is because leadership provides a better platform for the nurses to realize their vision and transform the health care system. The public does not view the nurses as being better leaders. On the other hand, the nurses do not commence their careers with the concept of leadership in mind. Every nurse is required to become a leader in their space (Kaihlanen, Hietapakka & Heponiemi, 2019). They need to be culturally competent leaders to help evaluate, implement, and design the ongoing reforms within the system.

To foster cultural competence in nursing, nurse leaders have to lead from the front. They need to take the responsibility of leading the rest of the team to understand and implement cultural

11

competence in nursing. As a leader, it's not right to conclude facts without having a clear understanding of the events and seeking opinions of other staff members from different backgrounds whose opinions might differ (Garneau & Pepin, 2015). To achieve success, nurse leaders should begin by first taking their team and staff members through the concept of cultural competency. It's best first to understand the concept and align with the organization's mission and vision before its implementation. The team should be educated and enlightened about what nursing's cultural competency meant (Loftin et al., 2013).

It should be understood that cultural competency is the process of developing a clear awareness of one's thoughts, existence, environment, and existence. The perception should negatively affect others or influence them in any way. Cultural competence helps demonstrate a better understanding of someone's knowledge and culture. It also helps one to respect the clients' cultural differences as well as to adapt to the client's lifestyle. With this information on the meaning of cultural competency, the team is now ready to take part in the process of implementing cultural competence in nurses (Reyes, Hadley & Davenport, 2013).

Creating Cultural Competence within the Nursing Organization

The first thing to consider when implementing cultural competency is to create a room for aesthetic awareness. The nurses, at this point, should first involve themselves in a self-examination. They should first examine their artistic, professional background. It will help them be in a position of understanding the culture of their patients. They should then create an insight into one's cultural healthcare values and beliefs (Loftin et al., 2013). It will help assess a person's level of cultural awareness. The other thing is to ensure that the patients are satisfied. In this case, the nurses will come up with different ways that will help them understand the patients. They will first understand the patients' cultural dimensions. It will help set a better platform and create a better relationship among the patients and the nurses. The nurse will be able to serve the patient better in a more professional way (Douglas et al., 2014). The nurses should also be able to explain some of the healthcare requirements to the patients whose native language is not English.

Research conducted in one of the hospitals indicated that most women suffering from cancer were shy; hence did not understand some concepts. Explaining some of the terms to patients will help the patient feel satisfied. Some people from the marginalized communities are not used to the western culture (Loftin et al., 2013). They view it as being harmful as they are used to herbals. Therefore, the nurses should inquire from the patients on an alternative healing method that they best prefer. The nurses should also understand some of the roles of men and women in a tolerant society. The male in some societies are the decision-makers, and therefore their decision should be respected by the nurses (Gallagher & Polanin, 2015).

There are four main strategies of cultural competence that can be used by nurses to enhance the quality of care includes Cultural preservation, Cultural accommodation, Cultural repatterning, and Cultural brokering, among other strategies (Reyes, Hadley & Davenport, 2013). Cultural preservation is a strategy that involves the use of cultural practices that are considered sound scientifically. A good example is when a nurse provides ample environment and Koran for a Muslim patient to play before going to the theater room. The other strategy, Cultural accommodation, occurs when a nurse supports the use of certain cultural practices by a patient or his family as long as they don't pose a risk to a patient's health. A good example is the use of acupuncture to treat pain management when dealing with a Chinese patient. Acupuncture is a Chinese cultural practice where thin needles are inserted in certain points in the body to balance energy and boost a patient's well-being.

The other strategy of cultural repatterning occurs when a culturally competent nurse uses therapeutic actions that are meant to influence a patient into modifying their current health behaviors, which are influenced by their culture, in order to achieve better health outcomes while respecting their culture. A good example is in a case where a nurse educates a patient on the negative impact of their cultural practice, such as taking herbs on health outcomes (Reyes, Hadley & Davenport, 2013). Lastly, cultural brokering involves the use of cultural competence and health science knowledge to negotiate or mediate between traditional health beliefs of a community and the provisions of the health care system (Loftin et al., 2013). A good example is the case of a nurse who finds a balance between the use of cultural practices as well as provisions of the healthcare system to stop the spread of infectious disease in the community.

Nevertheless, various barriers can hinder the application of these strategies. One of these is the lack of the resources required to make a particular strategy or cultural practice a success. For instance, hospitals may not have the needles to perform acupuncture on a patent. Another limitation is the time required to apply a particular strategy or practice (Garneau & Pepin, 2015). For instance, there may be no sufficient time to allow a Muslim patient to pray before a surgery that is deemed urgent and which could put the life of a patient at risk. Another limitation is the health risk factors involved with a strategy or practice. For instance, brokering between certain cultural practices and the provision of the healthcare system could put other members of the society at risk (Reyes, Hadley & Davenport, 2013).

Nursing Implications

Cultural competence is important in nursing practice as it ensures that nurses are able to deliver culturally sensitive care to the patients they attend to. It is important for nurses to have a good understanding of the cultural background of the patients that they serve. Community health nurses attend to patients and groups of people with varying cultural backgrounds (Kratzke & Bertolo, 2013). Cultural competence in nursing ensures that nurses embrace the culture and traditions of the diverse communities that they serve and, as a result, find ways to provide care

14

within a patient's culture and beliefs. Besides, nurses are able to get an understanding of the unique healthcare needs of the population that they serve and how this is affected by their cultural practices (Loftin et al., 2013).

A culturally competent nurse is the one that acknowledges the existence of cultural values, puts into practice and assessment of cross-cultural relations, discovers an impact of the differences in culture, and also provides unique cultural needs. Furthermore, the nurse should also be able to offer services that meet the needs of different cultures (Garneau & Pepin, 2015). In my nursing practice, I had encountered many situations whereby high levels of cultural competence are required. For instance, the case of an elderly Irish woman who was hospitalized, and she had to undergo surgery. She complained of pain to her family members, but she could not confess that to us since the Irish culture required women to hide the pain. The family members requested that the surgery date be brought up, but since the physician was unaware of this culture, he declined their request. The patient's condition deteriorated, and she died later during the surgery. If there were a culturally competent nurse, he/she could have intervened, and maybe the situation would have been controlled (Kaihlanen, Hietapakka & Heponiemi, 2019).

Therefore, it is advisable for nurses to be culturally competent, which will help them respond to the cultural huge healthcare demand of people from different cultures. Nurses can help reduce the health disparity and ensure quality healthcare to all people only if they help propel the health industry towards cultural competency (Gallagher & Polanin, 2015). The diverse healthcare environment is increasing, and therefore it is very critical for nurses to fully adapt to all cultural standards and implement them as required. Therefore the healthcare settings should introduce policies whereby a nurse can specialize in the specific cultural field, and this will result in a future culturally competent nursing practice (Garneau & Pepin, 2015).

15

Conclusions

In conclusion, cultural competence in the field of nursing has been described as the ability of healthcare providers to provide services that respect and also recognize the social beliefs and cultural practices of their patients. In this regard, a culturally competent nurse is the one that acknowledges the existence of cultural values, puts into practice and assessment of cross-cultural relations, discovers an impact of the differences in culture, and also provides unique cultural needs. Cultural competence is thus an essential component and element in nursing practice because it helps in striking a balance between culture, socio-economic issues, and political issues of nursing. Moreover, the states that have developed a curriculum for the training nurses is a step towards having a culturally competent nursing workforce. This is not only important for the nurses, but it will also contribute to improving the patient's outcome by increasing patient safety through the equity provision of care for all the patients while respecting the cultural differences between the nurses and the patients.

References

Almutairi, A. F., McCarthy, A., & Gardner, G. E. (2015). Understanding cultural competence in a multicultural nursing workforce: Registered nurses' experience in Saudi Arabia. *Journal of Transcultural Nursing, 26*(1), 16-23.

Cai, D. Y. (2016). A concept analysis of cultural competence. *International Journal of Nursing Sciences, 3*(3), 268-273.

Douglas, M. K., Rosenkoetter, M., Pacquiao, D. F., Callister, L. C., Hattar-Pollara, M., Lauderdale, J., ... & Purnell, L. (2014). Guidelines for implementing culturally competent nursing care. *Journal of Transcultural Nursing, 25*(2), 109-121.

Gallagher, R. W., & Polanin, J. R. (2015). A meta-analysis of educational interventions designed to enhance cultural competence in professional nurses and nursing students. *Nurse Education Today, 35*(2), 333-340.

Garneau, A. B., & Pepin, J. (2015). A constructivist theoretical proposition of cultural competence development in nursing. *Nurse education today, 35*(11), 1062-1068.

Jeffreys, M. R. (2016). *Teaching cultural competence in nursing and health care: Inquiry, action, and innovation.* Springer Publishing Company.

Kaihlanen, A. M., Hietapakka, L., & Heponiemi, T. (2019). Increasing cultural awareness: a qualitative study of nurses' perceptions of cultural competence training. *BMC nursing, 18*(1), 1-9.

Kratzke, C., & Bertolo, M. (2013). ENHANCING STUDENTS'CULTURAL COMPETENCE USING CROSS-CULTURAL EXPERIENTIAL LEARNING. *Journal of Cultural Diversity, 20*(3).

Loftin, C., Hartin, V., Branson, M., & Reyes, H. (2013). Measures of cultural competence in nurses: An integrative review. *The Scientific World Journal, 2013.*

Montenery, S. M., Jones, A. D., Perry, N., Ross, D., & Zoucha, R. (2013). Cultural competence

   in nursing faculty: A journey, not a destination. *Journal of Professional Nursing*, *29*(6),

   e51-e57.

Reyes, H., Hadley, L., & Davenport, D. (2013). A comparative analysis of cultural competence in

   the beginning and graduating nursing students. *ISRN Nursing*, *2013*.

Sharifi, N., Adib-Hajbaghery, M., & Najafi, M. (2019). Cultural competence in nursing: A

   concept analysis. *International journal of nursing studies*, *99*, 103386.

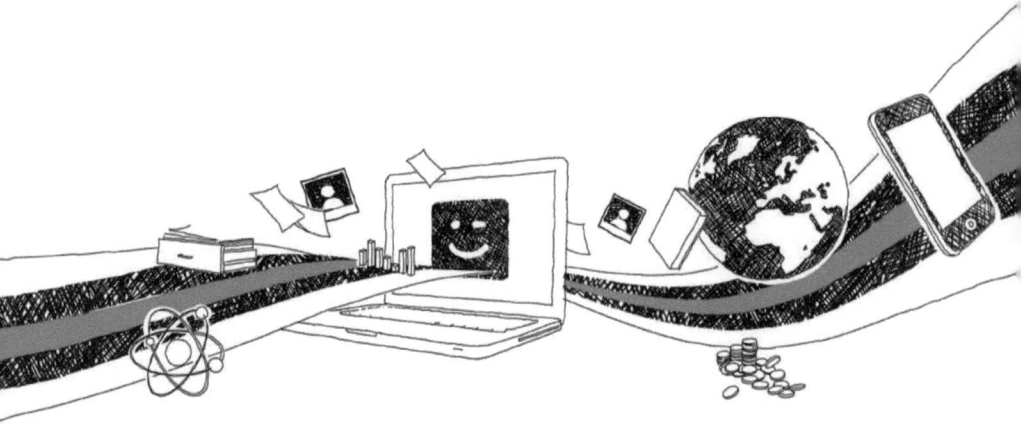
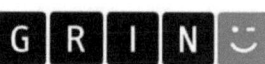